T0001488

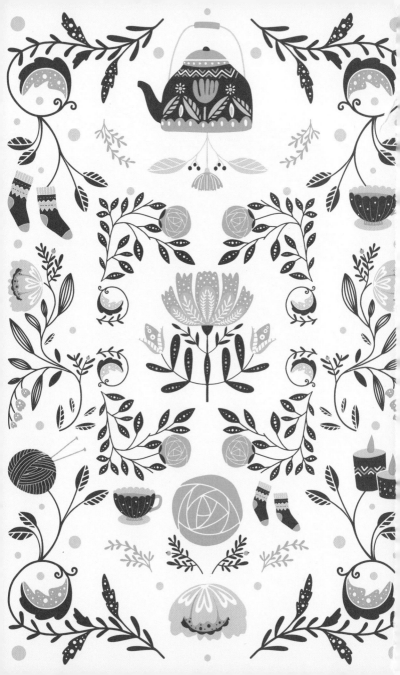

HYGGE
SIMPLIFIED

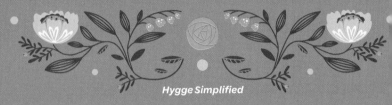

Hygge Simplified

13-Digit ISBN: 978-1-64643-214-1
10-Digit ISBN: 1-64643-214-2

This book may be ordered by mail from the publisher. Please include $5.99
for postage and handling. Please support your local bookseller first!

Books published by Cider Mill Press Book Publishers are available at special discounts
for bulk purchases in the United States by corporations, institutions, and other
organizations. For more information, please contact the publisher.

Cider Mill Press Book Publishers
"Where good books are ready for press"
PO Box 454
12 Spring St.
Kennebunkport, Maine 04046

Visit us online!
cidermillpress.com

Typography: LiebeErika, Looking Flowers, Omnes

All vectors used under official license from Shutterstock.com.

Printed in China
2 3 4 5 6 7 8 9 0

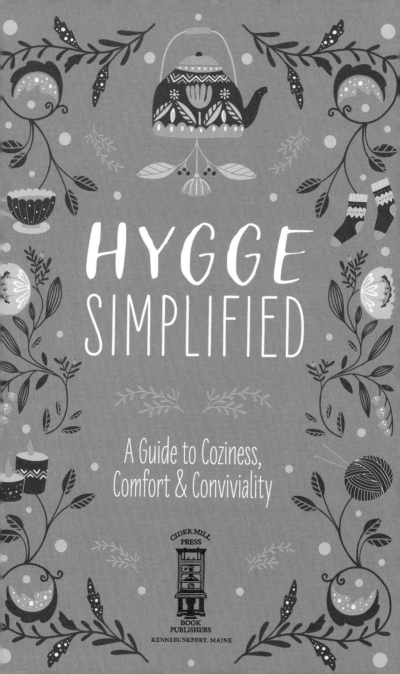

HYGGE
SIMPLIFIED

A Guide to Coziness,
Comfort & Conviviality

CIDER MILL
PRESS

BOOK
PUBLISHERS
KENNEBUNKPORT, MAINE

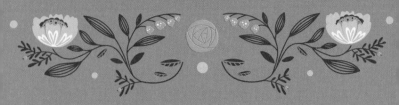

CONTENTS

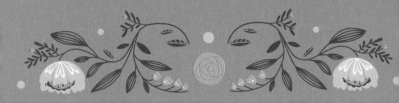

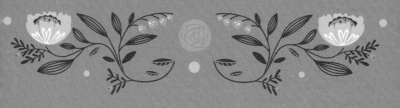

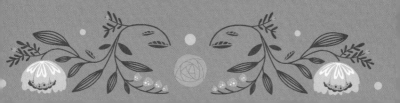

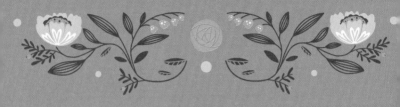

INTRODUCTION

HYGGE
("HOO-GA")

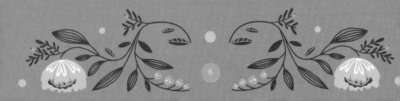

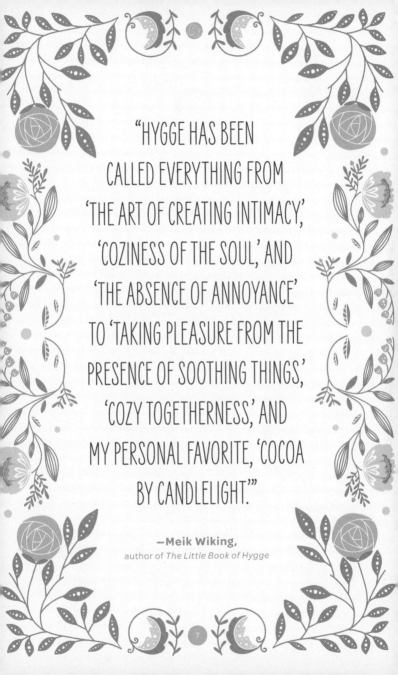

"HYGGE HAS BEEN CALLED EVERYTHING FROM 'THE ART OF CREATING INTIMACY,' 'COZINESS OF THE SOUL,' AND 'THE ABSENCE OF ANNOYANCE' TO 'TAKING PLEASURE FROM THE PRESENCE OF SOOTHING THINGS,' 'COZY TOGETHERNESS,' AND MY PERSONAL FAVORITE, 'COCOA BY CANDLELIGHT.'"

—Meik Wiking,
author of *The Little Book of Hygge*

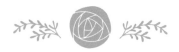

Hygge is very much in the news these days, especially in the wake of the global pandemic that kept so many of us shut away in our homes for over a year. You may have read online articles about it, seen videos, found hygge books in stores in the "Lifestyle" section, or heard your friends going on about it. But this Danish idea means more than just "happiness." So what is it really?

The concept of hygge originates in Denmark, which may not be surprising when you learn that Denmark is consistently rated as one of the happiest countries in the world (as are the other Scandinavian nations). But why would the birthplace of this idea be in a region known for its long, cold, and dark winters? What's up with all those happy Danes?

As you probably noticed from Meik Wiking's quote on page 7, hygge is not a word that can be translated easily into a single word, idea, or concept. It's more like a feeling than an idea, and different people will feel it in different ways. Hygge is very personal in that respect. At its heart, hygge is about enjoying the comforts of our home or space, cozy things, our treasures, our safety, and the familiar. It's about having a "safe space," in a very real sense, and of either reveling in that place by oneself or sharing it with a few good friends or family members.

It might be a nice dinner shared with the family or having your two best friends over for wine and conversation. It might be snuggling up under a blanket on a cold winter day and savoring a mug of tea and a good book. It might be making popcorn and enjoying a movie with your significant other. It definitely could be making a fire on a January night and basking in its toasty warmth.

Do you like lighting your home with candles at night, or maybe with soft mood lighting? Do you have a favorite armchair to curl up in? Do you have a beloved pet that sits on your lap while you read or watch television? Do you love baking cookies? Do you bask in the aroma of freshly brewed coffee? All of these things are hygge. So now you're probably getting a sense of why there isn't one good translation or definition. Hygge will mean different things to different people. It has as many meanings as there are people who enjoy it.

And you're probably also getting a sense of why this concept is so popular in Scandinavian countries. What can a cold, snowy, stormy night do against pleasures like these? Hygge is about love and life, and warmth and comfort, which is why it's become a common practice in Denmark, and in other places now. Regularly indulging in its principal pleasures contributes to one's overall well-being and creates emotional satisfaction. That so many Danes seem to engage in this practice explains a lot about why their nation is so happy.

Now, you might be thinking that this all sounds great, but you're not Danish (or even European), you don't live in a cold area, and hygge seems like something that costs a lot of money and requires a lot of effort. The good news: none of that is true! Hygge is not about being warm in cold weather, nor does it require lavish expense. In fact, spending a lot of time and money kind of defeats the point, which is to be happy with simpler pleasures. Often, the more rustic and homemade, the better! And while it might seem like hygge is best enjoyed at the holidays or in cold weather, it can be indulged anywhere, at any time of year.

The idea is to take yourself away from your worldly cares, even if only for a short time, and treat yourself to something that is just yours, or just for a small group of you and your closest friends. Hygge can also be experienced cheaply and entirely on one's own, whenever you want.

Hygge is really about creating an atmosphere of comfort for yourself, whether that be at home, at work, or in the outside world. It's about enjoying the moment and not feeling bound by obligations. Hygge is not something you *do* so much as something you feel and experience. That feeling of security and comfort becomes something you can step into as you return home and shed the outside world and its cares, even if only for a few minutes at a time.

This little book will introduce you to the wonderful world of hygge and show you how to bring these ideas into your own life, experiencing a little more comfort, happiness, and coziness as you do.

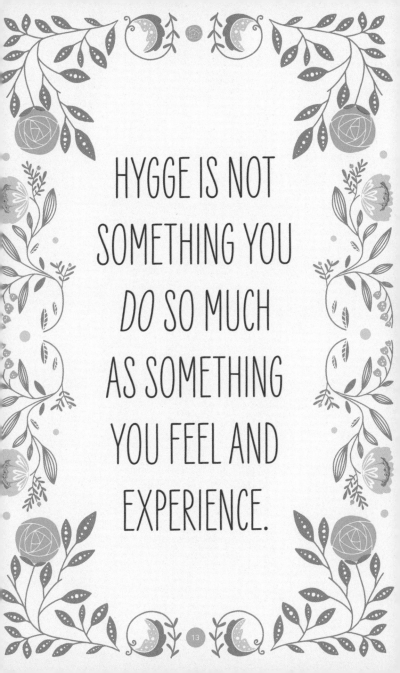

HYGGE IS NOT SOMETHING YOU *DO* SO MUCH AS SOMETHING YOU FEEL AND EXPERIENCE.

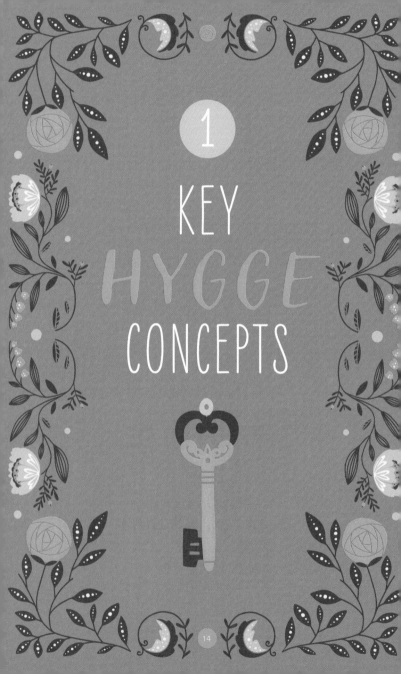

1

KEY
HYGGE
CONCEPTS

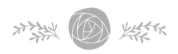

So what are the qualities of hygge? Here are some concepts to keep in mind as you begin to think about creating a special space that's all your own, or for you and those closest to you.

THE SETTING

The way that your space is organized is central to the whole experience. The lighting, the atmosphere, and what you choose to put in the space will all enhance your hygge feelings and make your space inviting and desirable. Personalize your surroundings exactly the way you want them.

FEELING SAFE

One of the main goals of the hygge space is to provide a little sanctuary from the cares of the world. So make sure that you can feel safe where you are. This also means that when you want to have some hygge time, you turn off your phone, ignore social media and the news, and give your attention to the here and now.

FEELING GOOD

Enjoy that tea or coffee, revel in those decadent little chocolates that you love, put on your favorite music, and do whatever makes you feel great. Hygge is about indulging in the things that bring you happiness and savoring the experience of simple pleasures at that moment. It's not about being elaborate or expensive.

SHARING

Hygge can be experienced on your own, but it's also a wonderful thing to share with others. That coffee is great, but it can be nice to have someone else to enjoy it with too. Does your family love those cookies as much as you do? Break them out and indulge together!

HUMILITY

Hygge is not about competition or spending lots of money. Its pleasures are simple, familiar, and, often, the more homespun, the better. Do you have a treasured blanket or stuffed animal from childhood that you won't part with? Maybe a vase that you made in a pottery class long ago that you're still proud of? These are definitely hygge, so delight in those simple objects.

THANKFULNESS

Being grateful for what we have, rather than what we think we want, is a natural part of hygge. And being grateful for the security around us and the space we've created for these moments is one of the best feelings we can have. A hygge moment is a lovely time to reflect on what you're thankful for.

COZINESS

Think of warmth, color, comfort, taste, and smell—all the details that make you feel good and secure. A soft blanket, the aroma of bread baking in the oven, and the glow of a candle are all very cozy and inviting. Often these feelings are most obvious during the winter months, when we can hear a storm outside and know that we have our own little corner of the world that nothing can touch. Coziness brings out gratitude and feelings of safety too.

FRIENDSHIP AND CLOSENESS

Hygge is at its best with others. Now, there's nothing wrong with having hygge time on your own, especially after a long day. But the chance to share the experience with family or friends can also be enriching and lovely. Hygge can be particularly good for introverts, who might not be thrilled about going to a noisy party, but would welcome inviting over one or two friends for an evening of wine, popcorn, cake, and movies. Hygge with others can be whatever you want it to be, and that's the beauty of it. You're not expected to throw a lavish party; simply bring yourself and a few comforts.

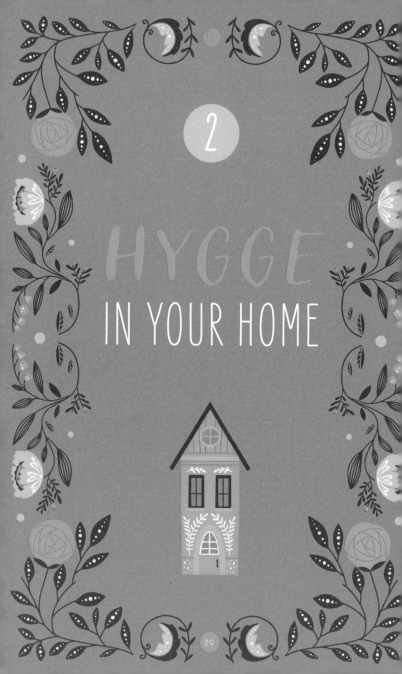

2

HYGGE
IN YOUR HOME

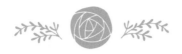

For Danes, home is really where the hygge is. They even have a special word for it (of course they do): hjemme hygge. Given that so much of hygge is about feelings of safety and security, it stands to reason that your home is the first and best place for you to enjoy hygge to the fullest.

Your home is where you'll probably have most of your hygge experiences, because you can tailor it exactly to what you want it to be. We all hope that our home is a safe haven against the world, and on a cold day, we may want nothing more than to stay home and curl up on the couch, eat some good food, and binge on a few episodes of our favorite TV show. Believe it or not, that's already a kind of hygge! You're seeking out a safe place to let your proverbial hair down and just be, and that's an essential part of hygge.

But what else can you do to make your home a more inviting place, where you can have that experience regularly or even daily? Wouldn't it be great to know that when you come home from work, you have your own little retreat that you've customized exactly the way you want it? Of course, you've probably already done a lot to personalize your abode; the suggestions in this chapter will help you add those extra little touches to make your home even cozier.

You may be worried that you have to do a lot of work or fork over a wad of cash to get things where they "need" to be. But it's not necessary to spend a lot of money to deck out your home. This goes against the spirit of hygge, anyway. You don't need the latest and most expensive decor; you need what's going to make you feel safe and happy. Using what you already have, plus a few small additions, can turn your home into a comfy haven that you'll never want to leave (one of the only downsides of hygge). Here are some suggestions.

CANDLES

Candles are essential for hygge. They are very popular in Denmark throughout the year, but especially in the winter months when the days are short. They provide a warm, atmospheric glow that always seems to perfectly light up a room. There's no need to go out and splurge on expensive candles (even tea lights will do the trick) or scented ones; Danes tend not to like scented candles too much, but if you do, that's also fine. Of course, you need to be careful, and never leave them unattended, but having a few well-placed candles in a room will make a big difference in its ambiance.

OTHER LIGHTING

Hot, blaring, bright lights are against the concept of hygge. Even if candles aren't really your thing, or you aren't able to burn them for safety reasons, think about how you can use dimmer lighting to help set a better mood. Maybe try turning off the main lights and using a small lamp placed in a corner? Or you could use LED tea lights, or even white Christmas lights. These are typically inexpensive and can provide great ambiance without any fire danger.

BOOKS OR OTHER MEDIA

Do you love to read? You probably already have (too) many books. And you may have them arranged on shelves in various places. Feel free to accent and showcase these volumes. Maybe you have an impressive CD collection that you won't get rid of (and if you do have one, that's great). Or maybe you own a collection of small objects or antiques that you're proud of. Be sure to display these in a way that makes them look good. A strategically placed candle or LED light may add a nice glow and flicker, for example (just be careful about an open flame near books). You can also accent stacks of books with little knickknacks (perhaps a small souvenir from a trip you took), a beautiful crystal, or a plant. These elements can add some dimension and warmth.

PILLOWS AND BLANKETS

Your couch probably already has a few pillows, and maybe you have a special blanket that you like to curl up under when the temperatures drop. If you normally only keep a blanket on your bed, try bringing it out to the couch once in a while. Again, pillows, blankets, and such don't need to be expensive or lavish in design; they just need to be things that make you feel comfortable.

NATURAL OBJECTS

Get a small bowl and fill it with a few items from the natural world. These could be pine cones, colorful fallen leaves, dried flowers, or some scented potpourri (though you'll need to change this out from time to time). A little centerpiece for your coffee table, or a display on a shelf between books, adds a nice touch.

ANYTHING VINTAGE

Wood, copper, ceramic—it's all great! Do you have any antiques at home? Things you've inherited? Something you picked up in a thrift store because you liked the look of it? All of these types of things are reminders of the past and can add an air of nostalgia to your home. Use what you already have on hand, especially if you have any kind of emotional attachment to it. Thrift and secondhand stores can be excellent sources of small, "rustic" items at very cheap prices. You can also use inexpensive pieces for DIY or upcycling projects. Check out crafting and painting tutorials on YouTube or blogs to get a sense of how you can transform something into your idea of hygge.

A FIREPLACE

You may or may not be lucky enough to have a fireplace in your home. There's a good chance that you don't. But if you do, and it's in working condition, it's well worth making use of it in the winter. Almost nothing says hygge like a crackling fire on a cold night. The sound of popping and hissing wood, whether in the stillness of the night or against the wind and the elements, while knowing that you are safe inside, is one of the best hygge experiences you can have. Just be sure that your fireplace is inspected and swept properly before using it for the first time. Dirt and other debris can collect and present a danger when flames are soaring up the chimney. If you don't have a fireplace, don't worry. You can still create that warm coziness with the other suggestions here, and it will make candles even more appealing.

A HYGGEKROG

Okay, this one isn't technically a must, but it's definitely nice if you can make it happen. A hyggekrog is a "nook," or a special place in your home that you can retreat to. It doesn't have to be an elaborately designed alcove, closet, or other location. It can be whatever makes you feel happy and cozy. It might be your favorite blanket and a pillow or two on the couch. It could be an old comfy chair that you adorn with said blanket and other comforting items. Maybe it's a breakfast table by a window that overlooks a nice yard or another scene. It's simply a place that makes you feel happy, and that lets you experience hygge whenever you sit there.

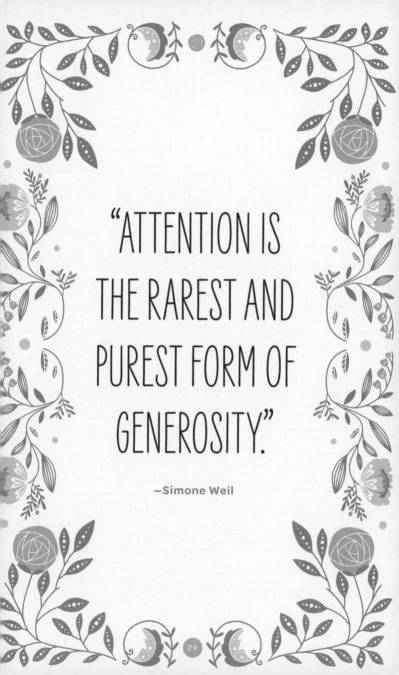

"ATTENTION IS THE RAREST AND PUREST FORM OF GENEROSITY."

—Simone Weil

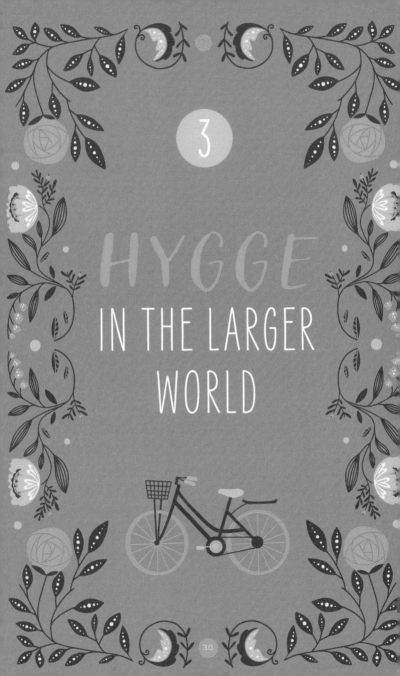

3

HYGGE
IN THE LARGER
WORLD

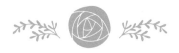

It's all well and good to talk about having hygge in your own personal space, which seems easy enough, but what if that's not an option for you? There might be any number of reasons that you can't decorate your living space the way you want it; you might be in short-term accommodation, or living in a dorm room, or dwelling with housemates with differing aesthetic ideas. Is it possible to capture some of that lovely hygge feeling in other places? Fortunately, the answer is yes! And if you can indulge in hygge experiences at home, it's perfectly fine to bring that feeling with you when you're out.

Here are some suggestions for how to bring the coziness and comfort of hygge with you almost anywhere you go.

AT ANOTHER HOME

If you can't set up your own living space the way you'd like right now, remember that hygge is not only about the setting. If you go over to a friend's home for an evening of hanging out, good conversation, snacks, and laughs, you can experience hygge just as well as you would at your own place. We're not talking about formal dinner plans here; hygge is all about being casual and comfortable. Having a few good friends can be essential to your experience, so reach out to them, if you're lucky enough to have them in your life. Your hygge place may be at your best friend's apartment, at least for a while.

OUTDOORS

While hygge is all about safety and comfort, there are times when being outside can bring out those same feelings. Maybe sitting on a beach, alone or with friends, and watching the waves roll in, is something that brings you immense joy. Bring a drink and a snack, and you have a lovely afternoon ahead of you that captures much of the hygge spirit. Do you like camping? Sitting around a campfire with a friend or two, sharing food and laughs, is certainly a hygge experience. Even going for a walk in the park can do the trick. It doesn't need to be elaborate. Going for a stroll at dusk and watching the evening mist drift in over the rooftops can be hygge, if you love it. Getting up to see the sunrise can be hygge. Maybe you have a local park bench that you like to sit in, just to watch the world go by for an hour. The natural world is very well suited to cozy, hygge experiences.

AT YOUR FAVORITE PLACE

Is there a café you love that makes the best coffee? Or a little restaurant tucked away on a quiet street that serves your favorite food? Do you have a bookstore where you can sit in a comfy chair and read for as long as you want? These are all great examples of hygge away from home. Seeking out these little refuges when you can will give you further chances to enjoy hygge beyond your personal space, or experience it when you can't have it in your own home.

AT THE OFFICE

Really? Sure, why not? While hygge at home is a retreat from the cares of the world, you can still bring some of that Danish magic into your job. As long as you're allowed to do so, making your work space friendlier and cozier for yourself is only going to help you when the days get long and drag, or you're under stress to get something done by a deadline. Can you dress up your cubicle a bit with reminders of coziness and comfort? Maybe a plant or some photos, or even LED tea lights? Can you organize a weekly tea and coffee break, where people bring sweets and share stories? Can you take your lunch and go for a walk in a nearby park? Be creative, and consider approaching your boss about ideas to "comfort up" the space a bit. Let them know it could very well improve morale and productivity, and they might go for it. You might transform your whole office into a hygge haven!

WHEN TRAVELING

Travel can be fun, and something you've been looking forward to for months. But it can also be stressful, and sometimes you might need a little reminder of home when you're far from it. This doesn't mean that you can ignite tea lights on an airplane or start a fire in your hotel room! But when you're out and about for business or pleasure, it's nice to bring something along that gives you that feeling of security and comfort you enjoy at home. Some people pack a favorite pillow or blanket, so that the hotel room doesn't seem as sterile and unfamiliar. (We all know how difficult it can be to sleep in a new hotel room on the first night.) Or maybe you have a little book of poetry that inspires you. Think about bringing something from home that will give you that sense of hygge.

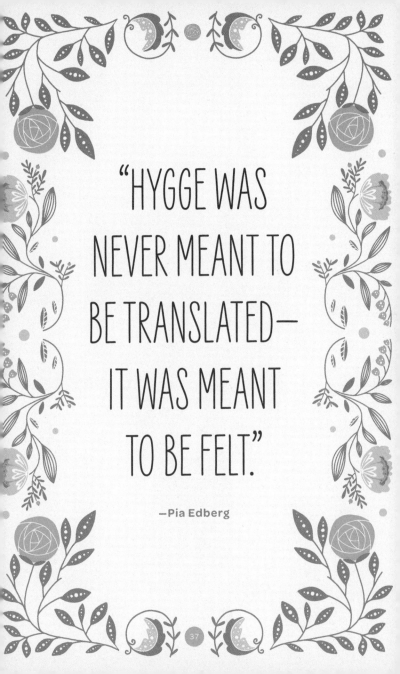

"HYGGE WAS NEVER MEANT TO BE TRANSLATED— IT WAS MEANT TO BE FELT."

—Pia Edberg

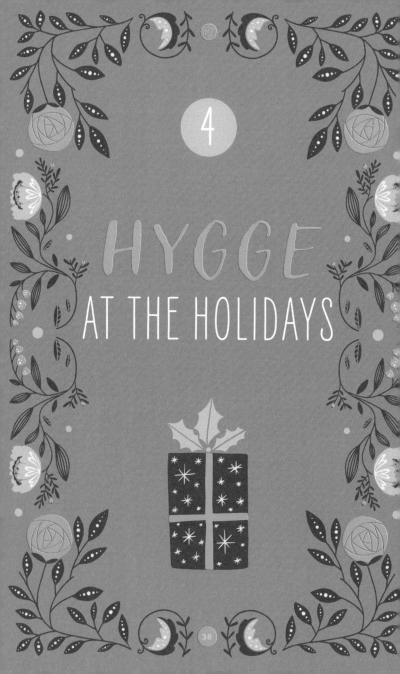

4

HYGGE
AT THE HOLIDAYS

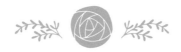

It probably seems pretty obvious, but hygge is tailor-made for the winter holidays. In Denmark, there's even a word for it: Julehygge. But "holidays" can mean any time that is special to you. It might well be the whole Christmas season, which in the Northern Hemisphere takes place in the colder, darker months. If you live in the Southern Hemisphere, your best hygge experiences might come in July and August. Maybe you're not interested in celebrating the December holidays at all. If you're a Hindu, Diwali and the time around it might be the perfect chance for some hygge. The same goes for Islam and Eid al-Fitr; in fact, breaking the Ramadan fast with family and friends could be a very hygge experience. Many modern pagans have eight celebrations throughout the year. But whatever you believe or don't believe, there are times when you may be more in the mood for some hygge than others, and that's fine. These suggestions are mainly for the months of December through February, but there's no reason you can't modify and adapt them to your own needs and wishes.

ACCEPT THE STRESS

This may sound contrary to the whole point of this chapter, but there's wisdom in adopting this attitude. For many (most?) people, the winter holidays can be a very stressful time. Rushing to make preparations, shopping for gifts and food, worrying about running up expenses, and so on are all very real concerns. It seems like every year we tell ourselves we're going to do things differently, but we keep falling back into the same stressed-out patterns. And you know what? That's okay. Hygge by definition stands in opposition to the stresses of the world, so in order to get to that space of coziness and safety, we may need to feel some discomfort first. The way many Danes see it, hygge must be put off until the preparations are done, which is what makes it more special when the time comes. We can't be in a state of hygge all of the time, or it wouldn't mean anything.

CUT DOWN ON EXTRAVAGANT GIFTS

One Danish trait when it comes to gift giving in a hygge mindset is to keep it as equal as possible. Someone who gives too many expensive gifts can be seen as boastful and acting as if they are superior. This might even make the receivers of these gifts feel that they owe something to the giver. If someone doesn't have much money, they may feel left out because they couldn't reciprocate in the same way. Presents are not competition. The best things in life aren't things, after all. Hygge is about the experience, not the price tag.

AIM FOR QUALITY OVER QUANTITY

Just as with gift giving, it's not about how elaborate your holiday meal is, how many decorations you have up, or how many people come to your party. A simple meal that everyone contributes to and enjoys together with genuine friends or close family members has just as much feeling and will be appreciated as much as some big, expensive bash. It should always be about the time well spent, the lively conversations, and the sense of goodwill.

CREATE AND CELEBRATE TRADITIONS

You probably already have a few family traditions that are trotted out every year during the holidays. Some of these may be great, and some may be terrible; there's always that one person who brings an awful food item that everyone has to pretend to like. (Insert the joke about the fruitcake that keeps being re-boxed and passed around every year.) The holidays are a perfect time to try introducing some new activities, especially those that are more aligned with hygge. Light some candles. Make a new holiday drink that everyone will enjoy (see page 59). Commit to trying some new foods. Play a silly game. Watch a movie together. All of these things can become new traditions if people take to them and they enhance the seasonal mood. Get creative and brainstorm with the others to see what might go over well. The goal is to come up with ideas that everyone enjoys, and yes, that's not always easy. Some work ahead of time will increase the chances that your get-togethers are fun and worthwhile for everyone.

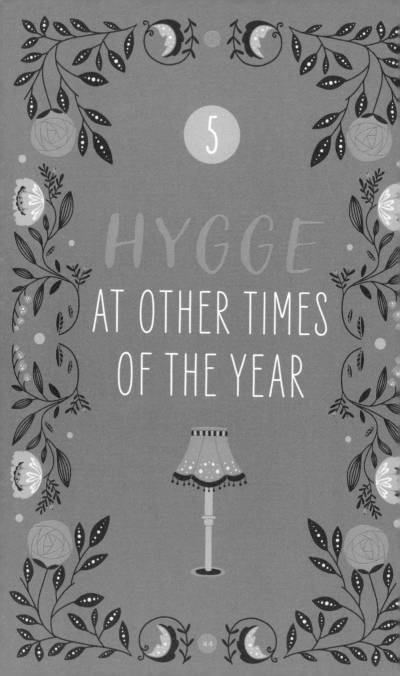

5

HYGGE
AT OTHER TIMES
OF THE YEAR

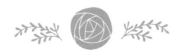

Hygge is typically centered on the northern winter holidays, so you might be wondering what you can do when those happy (if stressful) days have come and gone, and the reality of the long slog of January sets in. It's no secret that people can feel down and depressed after a busy and exhausting holiday season, but self-care during this time is, if anything, even more important. January and February can have very short days in some northern regions, weather that makes you never want to get out of bed, and all sorts of lovely things like cold and flu bugs flying around. If you're having a case of the after-holiday blahs, there are many things you can do to keep the feeling of hygge going in the months ahead. Try out some of these suggestions, and see if they can help you keep the spirit of hygge alive all year round.

KEEP THE LIGHTS ON

In the darker months, candles and mood lighting are even more essential. Nice lights don't have to end with the holidays! Keep a stash of inexpensive candles on hand to light your way when you're in the middle of February, and spring seems like a distant hope. Conversely, some gentle summer candlelight can only enhance the mood. Flameless lights work too, of course.

TV NIGHTS

This is one of the most obvious choices, and it's something you can do on your own or with family and friends. We've all become much more acquainted with binge-watching shows during the COVID lockdowns, so having time with yourself or with family to enjoy a cherished film or a favorite TV series can be just the thing at any time of the year. Make popcorn, break out your beverage of choice, and dive into your favorite movie or TV experience. Make it a weekly event, or even several nights a week, if you can.

POTLUCK DINNERS

One of the great things about having friends over for dinner is the chance for everyone to contribute. This takes all the pressure off of one person who has to play host and provide all the food (unless you really enjoy doing that; then, by all means, do). Come up with themes: a cuisine, one kind of food made in different ways, an all-snack meal, etc. Get creative and see what you can all think of. In the summer months, this might be a barbecue or a picnic. Just be mindful of people's dietary restrictions and needs. It's best not to invite your vegan friend to an all-steak bash, for example. And a gluten-intolerant person won't enjoy your spread of fine French pastries.

INEXPENSIVE WINE TASTINGS

If wine is your thing, it's possible to host tastings that won't break the bank. Invite a few friends over, and have each person bring one bottle of something to share. Again, this can be organized in many ways: by varietal, by country of production, by year, bargains under $15, etc. This is a great opportunity to try out new wines you may never have had or even heard of before. If wine's not your thing, beer is good, and so is cider. You can use nonalcoholic drinks too. A tasting of cordials, juices, or even teas can be a fun way to spend an evening.

BOOK CLUBS

Do you love mysteries? Or maybe epic fantasy and science fiction? Why not have a few friends all agree to read the same book and get together for a chapter-by-chapter discussion, with drinks and snacks? Everyone could commit to, say, reading one or two chapters a week, which should be manageable. As you discuss the story, you may discover things about the plot and characters that you hadn't thought of before and gain new insights into the work. Book clubs work for fiction and nonfiction—pretty much any book you'd enjoy talking about with others. Book clubs can also meet remotely online, so you can have friends in other parts of the country or world join in. Make it a bring-your-own-snacks-and-drinks event and enjoy the company of people from far away.

WALKS AND BIKE RIDES

If weather permits (or even if it doesn't), grab a friend or two and get outside. You can go for a walk in the country, or explore a part of town you've never seen before. Is there a museum or art gallery with a new exhibition? Go check it out! This can be fun for a small group or even for taking yourself on a "self-date." Likewise, if you have a bike, commit to getting out on it a little more, on your own or with others. It's great exercise and might give you some hygge moments that you'll remember for a long time. The Danes love their bikes and ride them everywhere. In Copenhagen, dedicated bike lanes are just as crowded as the streets with cars, if not more so, which is a lovely thing to see.

STARGAZING

Why not go out at night and look up at the sky? Gather a few friends or family members and go someplace where you can get a great view of the night sky. Obviously, this works much better away from the bright lights of the city, but if you're fortunate enough to have access to a place that's a little darker and more rural, this can be a great way to have a lovely experience. Try it out at different times of the year, and see how the night sky changes over the months. As always, bring a snack or some drinks (non-alcoholic, if you're driving), and let the evening become a memorable one.

GOSSIP NIGHTS

Okay, this doesn't technically have to be about gossiping; treat it as a great chance to catch up. Sit down with some snacks and a few drinks and see who's been up to what. This kind of activity can be done in a small group in person, or online via video; the online option is especially great if you're trying to reconnect with people who live far away from you. Again, you can have a theme, or it can be a general gab-fest. What's that pen pal in Australia been doing? Here's a chance to find out!

GAME NIGHTS

We all love games, and having a regular night set aside for board games is something that almost everyone will look forward to each week or every few weeks. Or maybe you're into role-playing games and want to get your D&D or Call of Cthulhu on! This is another activity that can be done in person or remotely, and it can be an ongoing activity. Brings snacks and have fun.

DO YOUR OWN THING

These suggestions prove that hygge is very often about forming and keeping deep connections with others, which only enhances the whole experience. But it may be that you're introverted, not very social, or just don't have a lot of friends or family at the moment. If so, you can probably come up with your own ways for how to do some of these activities. There's nothing wrong with making your favorite food and curling up with a good book on your own. That kind of self-care is just as important.

And when it comes to socializing, you might be even keener on having online get-togethers than in-person ones. The good news is that hygge often works best when it's one-on-one, or a small gathering of three or four people, which is a "people number" that most introverts do very well with. Introverts tend to get exhausted at large parties, but an evening of food and drink with two friends with whom they are deeply connected can be one of the best things on offer.

You are no doubt well aware of your own likes and dislikes, so tailor your hygge experiences to the way you want them. These suggestions are just that, and you can no doubt create your own activities that match your interests. Be creative, and be willing to try new experiences, and you'll probably come up with at least a few ways of connecting that embody the spirit of hygge.

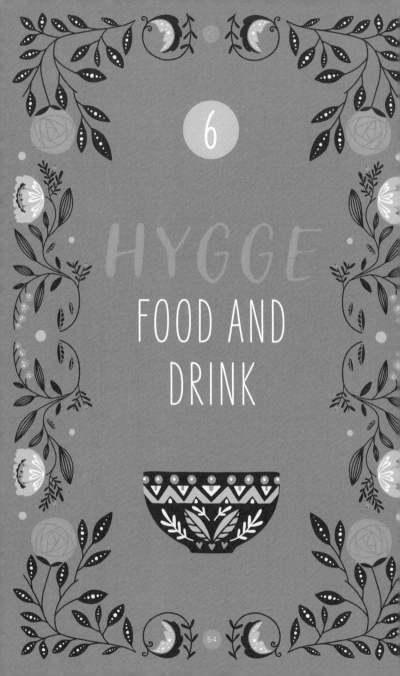

6

HYGGE

FOOD AND
DRINK

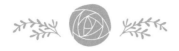

Food and drink can be an essential part of hygge. However, you don't need to go out of your way to make elaborate foods to bring to your hygge experience, unless you really want to. When the whole point is coziness and ease, comfort foods can be some of your best choices. You may already have a lot of these, and you can pick and choose whatever is best based on your mood. Do you have any childhood favorites that you still sometimes crave? A simple peanut butter and jelly sandwich can absolutely be hygge if it brings you happiness and nostalgia. Hot chocolate? Most definitely! With a few marshmallows floating on top? Even better!

But in the middle of the summer, a hot, warming drink might be the last thing you want. Do you like iced coffee or iced tea?

Those can be great alternatives, as can fizzy drinks and your favorite juice or smoothie. Changing your foods through-out the year is a great way to stay more in tune with the passage of time. You might even want to try eating seasonally for your hygge moments: eat only those foods that are in season in that time of year. This will give you a greater appreciation for what brings comfort during each season, as well as harkening back to much older days, when we couldn't get foods on demand. Of course, some foods, like chocolate, are fine at any time of year. This is a fact.

In short, there's no rule about how simple or elaborate your hygge foods need to be. Just go with what you enjoy and don't worry about whether or not you're doing it "right." If you enjoy a big plate of pasta or a bowl of popcorn, you're doing it right. Be sure to remember that the point of hygge is to savor the moment, indulge a little, and create spaces and times that are just for you and those closest to you.

If you'd like to sample some variations on your usual favorite drinks, try the recipes on the following pages.

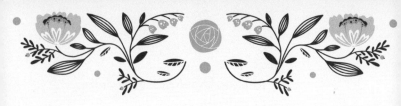

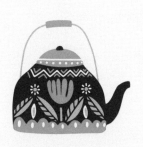

HYGGE
DRINK RECIPES

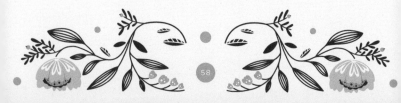

COFFEE

Coffee was probably introduced to Scandinavia from trade with the Ottoman Empire in the sixteenth century. But you might be surprised to learn that it wasn't very popular at first, at least not with the king, who saw it as a danger to public order and well-behaved citizens (it must have been all that caffeine). Coffee was heavily taxed and, at times, even banned to discourage people from drinking it, but its popularity grew over the centuries until it was fully legalized in the early 1800s. And coffee drinkers have never looked back! The Swedes even have a special term for the coffee break, fika, which is a whole world unto itself.

These days, we pretty much take coffee for granted. Arguably, it's the drink that runs the world, so the idea of using it as a way to slow down seems more than a little subversive. Of course, some people have issues with caffeine and can't drink it. That's no problem; there are many outstanding decaffeinated coffees that can be used as substitutes in these recipes, whether you're using a coffee pot, a drip, pods, an espresso machine, or any other method. Or maybe you don't like the flavor of coffee. That's okay too! When enjoying your hygge moments, you can drink tea (more on tea in a bit) or whatever other beverage you prefer.

But assuming that coffee is your drink of choice, here are a few recipes that go beyond everyday coffee and offer a little more in taste and sensation. Your regular coffee is just fine, of course, but these are some new ideas to add a little variety to your daily drink.

CARDAMOM COFFEE

Originating in India, cardamom is a popular spice in baked goods, but it works equally well in coffee. Various cultures (Turkish, Ethiopian, Indian) have enjoyed cardamom in their coffee for centuries, and it makes a lovely addition to any cup. Cardamom coffee can be made in whatever way you prefer to make coffee.

If you grind your own beans, crush open 2 to 4 cardamom pods (to taste) and remove the seeds inside. Discard the pods. Add these seeds to the beans before grinding; alternately, add up to ⅔ teaspoon ground cardamom to the mix, especially if you buy ground coffee. Use a French press, the pour-over or drip method, or whatever technique you prefer.

You may need to adjust the amount of cardamom to taste the first few times; a good place to start is one pod per cup to be served. Cardamom can disappear a bit into the stronger coffee flavor, so keep that in mind, and add more as you need and like.

CINNAMON COFFEE

Cinnamon is another spice that works well in almost any hot drink: coffee, tea, cider, etc. It's spicy, warming, sweet, and surprisingly good for you! Try adding some to your coffee for a nice twist on your usual cup.

You can add 1 to 2 teaspoons ground cinnamon to 2 cups coffee beans or 10 tablespoons ground coffee and prepare as usual, adjusting for taste, with 1 or 2 teaspoons per pot of coffee made.

Alternately, you can set a cinnamon stick in your coffee mug (as you would with hot cider) and just let it sit, giving you a nice, subtle warming flavor.

MOCHA COFFEE

Chocolate and coffee, who doesn't love that combination? Make your hygge drink an extra treat once in a while with this recipe.

The simplest way to make mocha coffee is to stir 1 tablespoon unsweetened cocoa powder into your mug of freshly brewed coffee. Add sweeteners or not as you like, and you're good to go!

OTHER COFFEE BLENDS

Have fun trying out other ingredients to jazz up your coffee. Try these alone, or mix and match and see what you like best.

Vanilla Coffee

Add 1 teaspoon vanilla extract per cup. Add to the grounds before brewing.

Bourbon Coffee

Add a splash of bourbon (or another spirit, such as rum) to your mug, if you want to live a little!

Nutmeg Coffee

Sprinkle a little nutmeg on top of your coffee in the mug.

Salted Coffee

Strangely enough, a pinch of salt can neutralize a bit of coffee's bitterness. Add ⅛ teaspoon (or less) to your ground coffee before brewing.

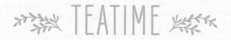

TEATIME

Does coffee make you cringe? Is tea your thing? No problem! There are plenty of alternatives to coffee when you're enjoying a hygge moment. Tea is an obvious substitute.

Whatever brings you happiness and comfort is what it's all about. Here are a few tea recipes that go beyond the usual. Again, if caffeine is your enemy, decaf tea and herbal teas are just fine (there's an herbal tea recipe below).

SPICY CHAI

Chai is an Indian classic, usually combining black tea, cinnamon, ginger, cardamom, cloves, black pepper, and other goodies into a heavenly mix that delights the senses and warms the body. Its spicy flavors are perfect on a winter day and go beautifully with sweet treats. While there are many great varieties that you can buy premade, it's fun to brew it up yourself and let those heavenly aromas fill your home. This tea can either have caffeine or not, as you prefer, and it can be made with hot milk (traditional), hot water, or a milk substitute. Use this basic recipe as a place to start, and vary it as you wish.

Makes 1 cup

1–2 whole cinnamon sticks

5–8 green cardamom pods

1 teaspoon whole black peppercorns

3–4 whole cloves

1–2 star anise pods (optional)

2–3 whole allspice berries, or ¼ teaspoon ground (optional)

2–3 fresh mint leaves, torn (optional)

2 tablespoons ginger root, grated or sliced, or ½ teaspoon ground ginger

3 tablespoons loose leaf black tea, or 3–4 black tea bags*

2 cups milk, dairy or plant based**

Sweetener to taste, if desired

* You can substitute decaffeinated tea for regular tea.

** Almond milk, oat milk, and soy milk are all good substitutes for dairy.

1 Add the cinnamon stick(s), cardamom pods, peppercorns, cloves, and, if using, the star anise, allspice berries, and mint leaves, to the bowl of a mortar (or cutting board) and use a pestle (or heavy pan) to crush a little. They don't need to be turned into powder. Just break them up enough to help release their flavors.

2 In a medium saucepan, add the crushed spices, 2½ cups water, and grated (or sliced) ginger and bring to a boil over high heat. Then reduce heat to medium-low and simmer for about 15 minutes, or until the mixture reduces by about one-third.

3 Add tea and milk and reduce heat to low. Cover and continue to simmer for 5 minutes to let the flavors blend.

4 Turn off heat and, still covered, let steep for 5 minutes, or longer for deeper flavor.

5 Add sweetener of choice to taste, if desired. Strain through a fine-mesh strainer into a teacup. Keep strained, cooled leftovers covered in the fridge for up to 3 days.

VANILLA TEA

Vanilla is a lovely flavor to combine with black tea or most herbal teas. This makes a great morning drink or a pleasant afternoon diversion.

The simplest way to enjoy this tea is to add ½ teaspoon vanilla extract to your mug after you've finished steeping your tea bag or tea ball, or however you prefer to make it. Alternately, you can buy vanilla beans, scrape the pods, and cut them into small pieces. Add them to a tin with your loose tea of choice and use the tea as you normally would. Use 3 to 4 beans per cup of dried loose tea. Vanilla sugar is a lovely alternative too; add to taste.

LEMON, GINGER, AND HONEY TEA

If you're in the mood for something without the black tea flavor, this recipe is just the thing. Enjoy it hot in the winter or cold in the summer for an invigorating and delightful drink that should go with just about anything you want to serve with it.

Makes 1 cup

1" piece fresh ginger root, grated or sliced

1 tablespoon fresh lemon juice

Honey, to taste

1 dash whiskey, to taste (optional, but nice)

1 Add the ginger to a small teapot or a large mug. Pour over 1 cup boiling water and let steep for 4 to 5 minutes. Add lemon juice. Strain the tea as you pour it into the mug.

2 Stir in honey and whiskey, if using.

With a touch of whiskey, this recipe resembles the classic hot toddy and is especially nice on a cold winter evening, or when you're sick. Of course, this is entirely optional. Alcohol is not necessary to enjoy this tea.

There are countless premade teas that you can buy, and if you prefer drinks like cider, flavored sparkling waters, etc., you can easily substitute whatever you want. Your perfect hygge moment may include a glass of your favorite wine, or simply some refreshing orange juice, or no refreshments at all. It's your time, and you get to decide how best to spend it.

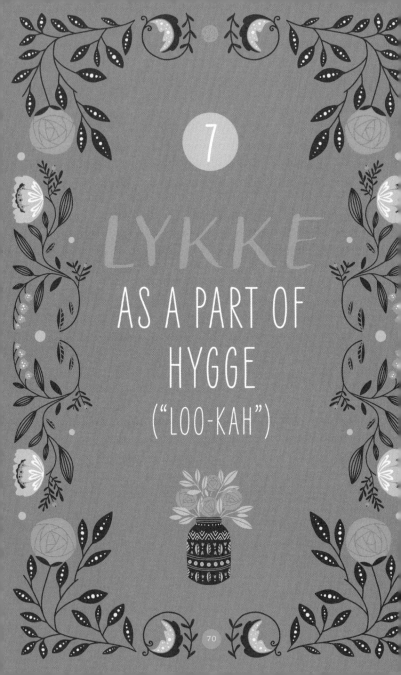

7

LYKKE

AS A PART OF
HYGGE
("LOO-KAH")

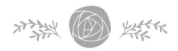

One of the main purposes of hygge should be to improve your life and thus increase your happiness. But what does that really mean? What is it to be "happy"? The funny thing about happiness is that almost everyone will give a different answer about what it means for them. So how can one Danish concept, lykke, bring everyone happiness? The answer is that it can't, or at least, it's not a cure-all. Think of lykke as a method, an attitude that you can use in your own life and circumstances. Combined with hygge, it can increase your sense of happiness and well-being.

As we've seen, the Danes are repeatedly listed as being among the happiest people on the planet. At first, this may seem obvious; a clean and modern country with excellent free health care, efficient public transportation, free education for everyone, and many other social benefits is bound to be a happy place. But it's less about those assets and more about the attitudes behind them. It creates a chicken-and-egg situation: Do these things make people happy, or do happy people create institutions that serve the public good, thus spreading around the happiness and letting it grow? It's a bit of both.

Remember, Denmark is a country with long, dark, cold winters, a lot of rain, and many days when you wouldn't want to go outside at all. And yet, the happiness factor is still there. We've seen the effect that hygge can have to counteract bad weather and bad days, but is it possible that something more is also present in many Danes' hearts and minds? Is lykke, their "happiness factor," something that anyone can tap into? The good news seems to be yes!

Meik Wiking is CEO of the Happiness Research Institute in Copenhagen, and he has studied and written a lot about Denmark's (and other countries') happiness. He is convinced that we can all bring this happiness factor into our own lives, wherever we might live. Most aspects of happiness are not exclusive to any one group or nation. They are available to us at any time, if we can be open to them and make some life changes here and there. What follows are some methods for you to cultivate a more Danish way of thinking about being happy, and bring extra happiness into your own life and the lives of your loved ones.

There's not one big secret or some magic pill that will take you to Happy Land, but as with hygge, doing a bit here and there will help you change how you look at some parts of your life and may well be the boost you need to begin feeling happier and more content.

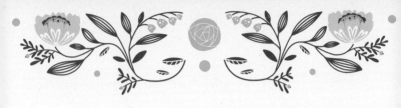

BEING
TOGETHER

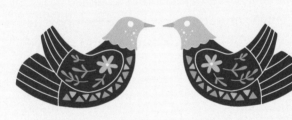

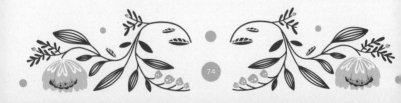

A key component of happiness is being with others of like mind, people who share our interests and enjoy being around us (hygge definitely includes and encourages this idea). These friends are there for bad times and good, and they give us a sense of belonging. Family is often the first place where this security can be found, but a chosen family can be an equally important alternative.

Remember that there's a difference between "loneliness" and "being alone." Having time to ourselves is very important, and most introverts crave this time as being essential to their mental and physical health. Being on your own and feeling happy are entirely compatible ideas. Loneliness, on the other hand, is the feeling of having no friends, no one to turn to (or not having someone often enough), and no one for support and encouragement. You can even have a large social circle and still feel lonely, if it seems like no one understands you or listens to you. Having a committed social circle, even if it's only a few people who really "get" you, is essential to happiness.

The Danes have a wonderful word for it: fællesskabsfølelse, which means something like "having a sense of community." In Denmark and Iceland, over 95% of people say that they believe they can rely on others in their times of need. That's a very powerful and reassuring feeling for people to have.

There's no doubt that loneliness is bad for our health. It can lead to depression or make existing depression and anxiety much worse. It can affect cognition, raise cortisol (stress hormone) levels, increase the risk of heart disease, disrupt sleep, and raise cholesterol levels. Clearly, this is not something we should take lightly. Loneliness is on the rise these days, and social media and pandemic isolation have only made it worse. So what can we do to help foster feelings of community and inclusion?

IF YOU'RE LONELY, TRY TO GET MORE IN TUNE WITH YOUR FEELINGS

Ask yourself what is wrong, what is missing, and think about ways you could fix that. Don't compare yourself to others; their story is not yours. Ask yourself how often you feel lonely, and if anything is triggering it. If so, what can be done to minimize those triggers?

TRY REACHING OUT

If it seems that everyone is ignoring you or doesn't want you around, that might not be the case. People get caught up in their routines, and it's hard to keep up with everyone. Try sending a few messages to people you haven't chatted with in a while. Often, people will get back to you and will be happy to catch up a little. It might be that they're feeling lonely too.

TRY TO SET UP SOME ONGOING TIMES TOGETHER

Whether a meetup is in person or via online video, email chat, or whatever, see if you can arrange a recurring time for you and a friend, or a few friends, to touch base with each other.

VOLUNTEER

One way to decrease your feelings of loneliness is to feel needed by others. If you can spare an hour or two a week to help a retirement home, an animal shelter, or anything you feel drawn to, it can be a great way to forge some new connections with other volunteers, as well as the people you're helping out. If you don't feel you have any reliable friends, try volunteering, and you might be amazed at how valued others come to see you.

CONSIDER HAVING A PET

Countless studies have shown the beneficial effects that come with having an animal companion. Of course, this is not going to be an option for everyone. You may not be able to keep a pet for financial reasons, or maybe you live in a place that doesn't allow them (all too common, unfortunately). In that case, if you're still fond of being around animals, try volunteering at a shelter, helping out with dog walking, or whatever else would get you into contact with more furry (or feathered, or scaly) friends.

CUT DOWN ON SOCIAL MEDIA

Ironically, these platforms that were supposed to "bring us together" often end up making us feel more isolated. We feel bad or even jealous when we look at all the cool stuff everyone else is doing, and we get the sense that we're not nearly as interesting. So of course, *that's* why we have no friends! The truth is that everyone likes to post their best selves on social media. Concentrate on a few good friends and don't worry about what the other 725 are doing. You probably don't really know most of them very well anyway.

CONSIDER SEEKING PROFESSIONAL HELP

There is no shame at all in seeing a qualified therapist to talk about your problems and concerns. If loneliness just won't go away, it may be time to talk to someone about it. Mental health is just as important as physical health, and you are right to take care of yourself.

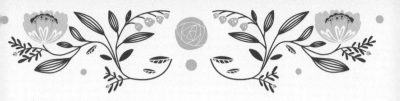

HEALTH

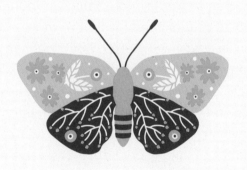

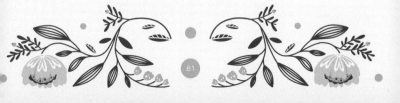

The link between health and happiness seems obvious, but it may surprise you how much they are connected. Unhappiness is linked to inflammation, higher rates of heart disease, more susceptibility to colds and flu, and shorter life spans, among other problems. Being unhappy is unhealthy!

The good news is that this relationship is something of a two-way street. The more your health improves, the happier you will be, but also, the more you can increase your levels of happiness, the more likely you are to have better health. Since so many of our modern health problems are aggravated by stress and worry, it stands to reason that if we can work to eliminate or diminish those problems, we have a good chance of upping our happiness levels and feeling better in both mind and body.

If you have health concerns, you should always consult your doctor or qualified health provider. But here are some simple steps you can take to improve your health right away. Other than the obvious ones like quitting smoking and cutting back on junk foods, of course!

GET MORE AND BETTER SLEEP

It's easier said than done, but we all know that sleep is vital to health. Chronic issues with poor sleep can indicate an underlying condition, and it's worth having that checked out. Take the time to actually get enough sleep. Try deep breathing, meditating, a hot bath before bed, and anything that will help you unwind. Since light from devices can be disruptive to our natural rhythms, power down the laptop and the phone an hour before turning out the lights, and let your mind disconnect from the day.

CUT DOWN ON SUGAR

This may seem like strange advice in a book about indulging in sweets for hygge, etc., but the point is to do everything in moderation. Have that chocolate cookie with your coffee, but don't have eight! Enjoy some cake with hot tea, but have just one piece. We tend to eat when we are upset, and sugar can be one of the most appealing tastes in those moments. Eat because it's a treat, not because you're trying to use food to escape. The same goes for alcohol. A glass of wine can be lovely; drinking the whole bottle yourself is not a good idea.

MOVE MORE

Take those stairs, ride your bike, use a standing desk. You may not be able to go to the gym four times a week, but getting your body used to the idea of doing some kind of movement every day will help you. If you work in an office, go out for lunch and make a habit of getting up once an hour or so to move, even if it's just to take a stroll around the building. Remember, the Danes are avid bike riders for a reason!

TRY MEDITATION

Meditation has been popular in Western countries since the 1960s, and it continues to grow in popularity and acceptance as more and more research confirms its benefits. One doesn't need to devote one's life to Eastern spiritual practices to take advantage of it. Try some simple mindfulness exercises for a few weeks (there are many guides to mindfulness on the internet). A calmer mind will translate into a more relaxed body, and getting rid of stress is one of the key strategies to improve one's health.

TRY A GENTLE MOVEMENT EXERCISE

Millions have found that yoga, tai chi, and qigong (among others) have definitely improved their health. You don't have to be super bendy to try yoga, or super coordinated to do tai chi. Qigong often involves just standing in place, but it can also be done while sitting. If none of these appeals to you, consider other gentle warm-ups and exercises, like pilates. Or, if you really want to embrace the Northern European lifestyle, check out Stádhagaldr (runic yoga), standing postures based on the ancient Germanic and Nordic runes. Another great option is Nordic walking, an exercise that is derived from skiing and trekking and uses poles. It engages more of the body and is considered an excellent workout for all ages.

Participating in one of these activities daily will almost certainly bring benefits. Exercise is a natural mood booster, but it doesn't have to be strenuous or vigorous if that's not your thing. It can (and should) be a part of your hygge moments, and thus should be something you enjoy doing.

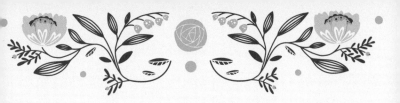

FEELING FREE

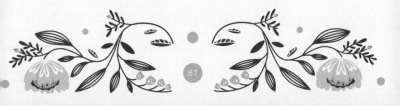

"Freedom" can mean anything from the status of the nation you live in and the rights of its people to how much time you have to yourself. And there is no doubt that with feeling free comes a good degree of happiness. The Human Freedom Index is an annual report that ranks nations by the level of their freedoms. As you might expect, nations like Denmark and Finland routinely score high, while China and Iran score low. The United States usually appears between fifteen and twenty on the list. Where someone is born and lives can have a profound effect on how free they feel.

Assuming that you are living in a relatively free country, here are some ideas to bring even more freedom into your life.

LOOK AT YOUR WORK SITUATION

If someone's work-life balance is out of whack, they can quickly find themselves devoting way more time to work than they would like. And this isn't just about the hours worked. It's about commute time, work taken home, Saturdays given up, etc. If you're feeling overwhelmed by your job, it might be time to evaluate what's important and what's making you unhappy. Money is important, and job security is important, but if you're only living to work, your happiness is going to plummet fairly quickly. And you'll have little or no time for hygge.

LIMIT SOCIAL MEDIA

This again! Studies have shown that while social media is meant to connect us, spending prolonged periods on these sites actually makes us feel worse, not only about the time we're wasting but also when we read about all of these wonderful lives everyone else seems to have. Keep in mind that many people are putting their best faces forward on these platforms, and their amazing updates are probably not indicative of what's going on in the rest of their lives. Take a break and read a chapter from a book instead. Change some of your social media time into hygge time.

MAKE BETTER USE OF THE TIME YOU DO HAVE

Going hand in hand with getting off social media, try to use the time you do have more effectively. Even recovering thirty minutes of "you time" a day will let you feel more in control and freer. If you can grab a hygge moment or two during this time, even better!

GIVE YOURSELF DEADLINES

So, you need to clean up your place over the weekend? Good, but get more efficient at it. Don't let it eat away your whole Sunday afternoon. Imagine that you have relatives coming over in an hour and you need to get it all done. It's amazing how much more efficient we can be under a deadline.

IF YOU'RE A PARENT, UNDERSTAND THE CHALLENGES

The so-called parental happiness gap is real. It's a measure of how parents compare their levels of happiness to the happiness of their friends who don't have children. And yes, more often than not, parents report feeling less happy due to the lack of time and freedom that being a parent can bring. But parents aren't doomed to unhappiness at all. Children in and of themselves are a great source of joy, and feelings of happiness often increase as the children grow up. In countries that have "communal parenting," i.e., regular help with children from grandparents and others, levels of parental happiness tend to be much higher. If, as a parent, you have others in your life who might be willing to help you, try seeking them out more often.

Freedom is a rather subjective concept. Some things in our lives that feel like constraints and traps may not be viewed that way by others. Using these suggestions as a guide, ask yourself what it is you need to feel freer. Having, say, thirty minutes of hygge time to feel relaxed and cozy a few days of the week might also increase your sense of being more in control of your time and the freedom to enjoy yourself.

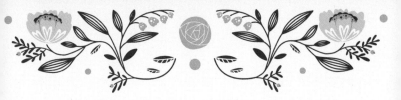

MONEY

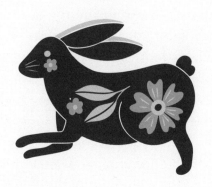

We've all heard that money can't buy happiness, and we tell ourselves this, even if we don't believe it. The thing is, it's true. Vast amounts of money rarely buy happiness for anyone. There is a concept in economics called the law of diminishing marginal utility. What this fancy term means is that a thing is always most desirable when we don't have it, and when we do, it can be great for a while, but the more of it we get, the less satisfying it is. Say you win the lottery and go out and buy a fancy sports car. It's awesome, but you don't just want one, so you get another, and then another. By your third or fourth car, they're probably not exciting anymore. This idea works even with simple things: the seventh cookie is not nearly as satisfying as the first one, and you'll probably just end up feeling sick. But what happens is that people buy more and more, desperately trying to re-create that initial euphoric feeling. And most often, they can't.

What money *can* buy is a greater feeling of security, and with it, freedom. And the desire for that security should not be diminished or dismissed. But all too often, people find themselves caught up in the trap that making more money is the ultimate goal, with no thought of what that might mean, or even what the point of it is. Because really, once you have all of your needs met and feel safe and secure and can do what you want and indulge in hygge at any time, how much more money do you need: $5 million, $10 million, $25 million, more? At some point, the diminishment sets in, and making money can become an empty goal in and of itself, almost like a pathological hoarding disorder. But assuming that you're not a multimillionaire, here are some ways of thinking about money that can contribute to your overall happiness.

BUY EXPERIENCES, RATHER THAN THINGS

Blowing money on a $3,000 watch produces very little long-term satisfaction, but spending the same amount on an amazing trip to Paris will give you a lifetime of memories from the experiences enjoyed there. Traveling to a new place or trying out a new sport appeals to our desire for novelty. These activities give us better value for our money because they speak directly to our emotions and sense of well-being. The Danish holiday custom of simpler gifts but great food and dinners is a lovely example of the value of experiences. Hygge is really all about the experiences, and often the simpler they are, the better.

LET BIG EXPERIENCES HAVE TIME TO GROW

If you're planning a trip, start planning it well in advance, so you have time for the anticipation and excitement to build. Having something to look forward to during those months will give you a sense of money well spent and an extra dose of happiness. You're spreading out that anticipation over a stretch of time, which gives the experience even more value.

IGNORE THE LATEST FADS

Do you really need the latest phone or gadget? The fancy coat? Probably not. Advertising agencies spend billions convincing you that you do, and the fear of missing out (FOMO) sets in. It's all manipulation to separate you from your money. Buy only what's meaningful to you.

ENJOY THE PROCESS

The plan may be to get the job promotion to make more money, but don't make that end goal your only focus. Take the time to appreciate what you're doing in the moment to achieve your goals. The journey is a big part of the process.

DON'T COMPARE YOURSELF TO OTHERS

Trying to keep up with your friends or colleagues is a surefire way to plummet into unhappiness. What's right for them is not necessarily right for you. Again, social media contributes to this yucky feeling.

IF YOU HAVE WEALTH, DON'T FLAUNT IT

Seriously, almost no one cares, and those who do are probably just resentful and envious.

ACCEPT THAT YOU CAN'T CONTROL EVERYTHING

You might be careful and frugal with your money, but things can still happen. Accept that risk is a part of life and that economies boom and contract, jobs come and go, and you may not always be in the same place you are right now. But being able to access those comforting moments is something you can always take with you, no matter what the outside world throws at you.

In general, a majority of Danes have responded to surveys saying that they expect to be happier in five years than they are now. This isn't about making more money, but rather a general cultural and societal expectation. Whether they're richer or poorer, they *expect* their happiness to improve as they grow and experience more of life. This is a great idea to live by!

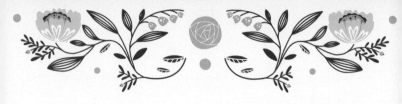

KINDNESS
AND TRUST

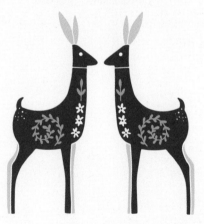

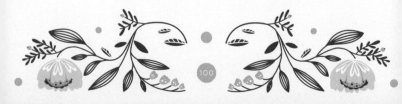

Having a community that you can rely on can be a considerable boost to overall happiness. Whether this is with your family, the neighborhood, or society at large, trust brings feelings of security and safety. Knowing that someone else has your back can give you peace of mind. So how do you build feelings of trust with others? Be trustworthy yourself, and treat everyone kindly and fairly. Once again, making others happy brings happiness to oneself, and being reliable and trustworthy will almost certainly open the door for others to treat you in the same way.

In 2015, the World Happiness Report noted, "A successful society is one in which people have a high level of trust in each other—including family members, colleagues, friends, strangers, and institutions such as government. Social trust spurs a sense of life satisfaction."

The Danes often display remarkable trust-worthiness. It's not at all uncommon for parents to leave their infants outside of shops and restaurants in their strollers. Yes, they are left unattended. No, almost nothing bad ever happens. It is such a deeply ingrained part of the culture that no one thinks anything of it. That's an amazingly deep level of trust! And while we might not have nearly as much trust where we live, we can work to improve trust with our friends, neighbors, and larger communities by being true, reliable, and kind. Here are some suggestions.

KEEP YOUR WORD

If you tell someone you're going to do something, do it. It's that simple. The more trustworthy you become, the more people will be willing to trust you. Conversely, don't make promises that you can't keep; be realistic, no matter how much you might want to be helpful.

LISTEN TO OTHERS AND GIVE THEM YOUR FULL ATTENTION

When someone is talking to you, listen and take a genuine interest in what they're saying. This builds rapport. They'll probably do the same for you, and if they don't, they might not be the right person to be friends with anyway.

ADMIT WHEN YOU'RE WRONG

It's the adult thing to do, and it will be far better for you in the long run. It shows that you have humility and are trustworthy. Trying to deny or cover up mistakes will get you nowhere. Never blame others for your own mistakes.

LEARN TO TRUST OTHERS MORE

This can be very hard if you've come from a background of being mistreated, abused, or betrayed, so be gentle with yourself on this one. You don't have to rush into anything. Try letting someone do something for you once in a while, no matter how small, to see how it makes you feel.

PRACTICE EMPATHY

Always be kind. Always try to see things from the other person's point of view. Resist the urge to be critical unless it's truly warranted. Read more fiction; interestingly, being able to empathize with fictional characters in a story has been shown to improve our own ability to empathize with others in real life. So when you settle in for a hygge hour with your tea and a good novel, you're also building empathy in the real world!

PRACTICE RANDOM ACTS OF KINDNESS

It can be fun to secretly do something that improves a person's day. There's no limit to what you can do: smile and say a friendly hello to everyone (and mean it). Send an email to a friend telling them you were just thinking about them and how much you value them. Take a friend to lunch, your treat. Compliment someone. Tip the overworked barista a little extra. Buy a small gift for your friend and give it to them just because. Buy a sandwich for a homeless person. Help without being asked. You can actively create mini hygge moments for others through kindness.

GET MORE INVOLVED WITH YOUR COMMUNITY

Are there simple things you can do for your neighborhood that would help others? This is a great way to build trust while acting kindly. In England, an anonymous individual nicknamed "The Free Help Guy" took this idea much further. He started asking people to email him when they needed help with something. The response was overwhelming, but he went to work on helping as much as he could and has done enormous good for many people, all for free. He's done everything from helping people find renters to trying to locate long-lost relatives to looking for donors for operations and transplants. He does it all because it makes him feel good, and it's probably safe to say that he's a lot happier than most people. Maybe some of your best hygge moments will come from being kind to others?

How we interact with other people has a lot to do with how happy we are. The Nordic countries in general have done a great job of building up levels of societal trust and a sense of the common good, so that people can get on with living their lives. But no matter where we reside, we can import some of those same ideas and practices into our own lives and make ourselves happier.

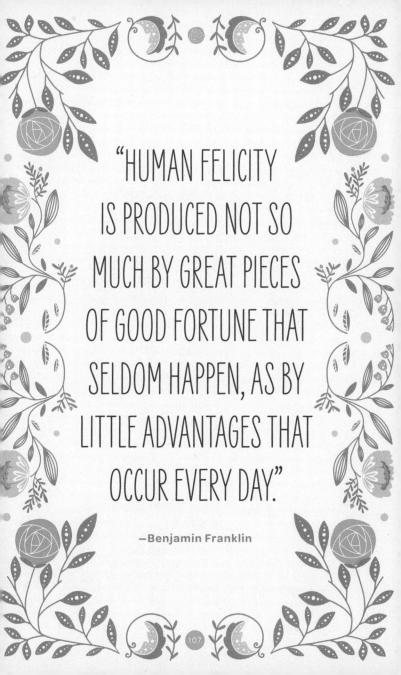

"HUMAN FELICITY IS PRODUCED NOT SO MUCH BY GREAT PIECES OF GOOD FORTUNE THAT SELDOM HAPPEN, AS BY LITTLE ADVANTAGES THAT OCCUR EVERY DAY."

—Benjamin Franklin

8

FINAL
THOUGHTS

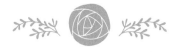

Taking a little time each day, or perhaps a few days a week, to slow down and do something personal, something that makes you feel safe and restored, is the essence of hygge. It need not be elaborate or expensive; all that matters is that it brings you a bit of joy and shelters you from the chaos and concerns of the larger world, if just for a while. A few moments of indulgence can do wonders for resetting and renewing.

While happiness is a goal of hygge, happiness is, as we've seen, a bigger idea, and one that the Danes approach both within hygge and on its own in the concept of lykke. These two ideas are intertwined, and cultivating one can help enhance the other.

You don't need to expend a lot of time or effort for hygge or lykke; you're not trying to stress yourself out to be happy! Using the ideas in this book, take some small, initial steps to increase your happiness and give yourself room to relax and breathe. A little time every day, or every few days, that's just for you can yield great results.

May this book be useful to you in becoming more happy, secure, and fulfilled!

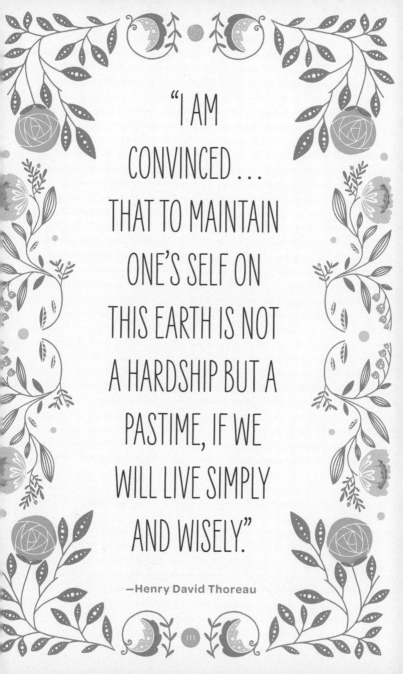

"I AM CONVINCED ... THAT TO MAINTAIN ONE'S SELF ON THIS EARTH IS NOT A HARDSHIP BUT A PASTIME, IF WE WILL LIVE SIMPLY AND WISELY."

—Henry David Thoreau

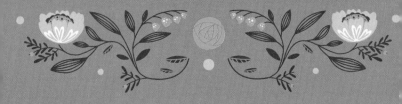

ABOUT CIDER MILL PRESS BOOK PUBLISHERS

Good ideas ripen with time. From seed to harvest, Cider Mill Press brings fine reading, information, and entertainment together between the covers of its creatively crafted books. Our Cider Mill bears fruit twice a year, publishing a new crop of titles each spring and fall.

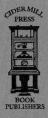

CIDER MILL
PRESS

BOOK
PUBLISHERS

"Where Good Books Are Ready for Press"

Visit us online at
cidermillpress.com

or write to us at
PO Box 454
12 Spring St.
Kennebunkport, Maine 04046

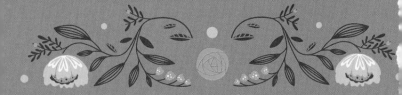

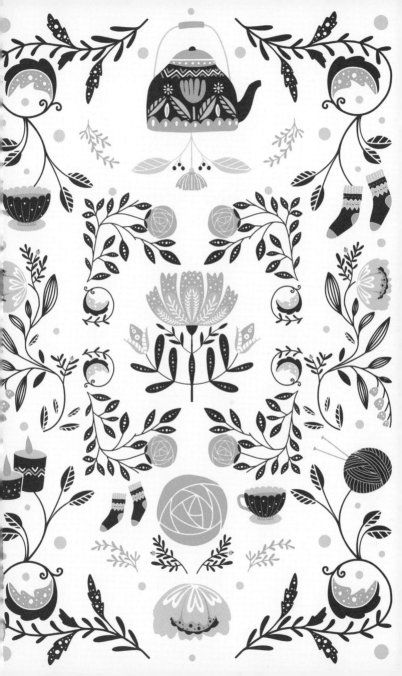

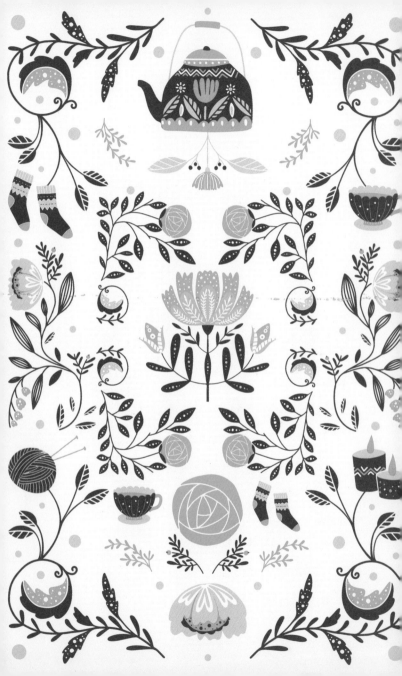